Ordering Information:

For details, contact *ganopeter@yahoo.com.au*

www.food4familiesproject.com

Printed in Australia

ACKNOWLEDGEMENTS

To the greatest gift I have been given,
The Father, the Son and the Holy Spirit.
My Lord, my God, and my King.
All the glory, and honor go to You.

To my wonderful family, my wife, Alma, and children,
Chloe, John-Paul, Nicole, Simon and Benjamin.
You are my inspiration, and I thank you for the joy
And the happiness you bring to my life.
It has been an amazing journey .

My dedicated friend Patsy. I am so glad you were
Johnny on the spot when my cardiac arrest happened.
Your calm manner got the CPR rolling
You helped save my life. Ever grateful.

The mystery nurse, Claire, who just happened
To be in the right place at the right time.
You coordinated the whole CPR exercise to perfection.
Thanks a million.

The paramedics, doctors, and hospital staff assisted
my recovery. A big thank you for your
professionalism and effort.

To my very talented and humble niece,
Rhea Mae Alibong, for your great work on
Editing and laying out this book.

Unmasking the Hidden Pandemic:
Hypothyroidism

"Reclaiming Your Health, One Step at a Time."

"Reclaiming Your Health, One Step at a Time" emphasizes the gradual and patient approach needed in your journey toward better health. It recognizes that healing is not instantaneous and that each step, no matter how small, is vital to the overall process. This phrase encapsulates the idea that managing hypothyroidism—or any health condition—is about making consistent, thoughtful changes over time, rather than expecting immediate results.

In your story, this could mean understanding that every action you take, whether it's adjusting your diet, changing your supplement routine, or incorporating new lifestyle habits, is a step toward improving your health. It acknowledges the ups and downs of the journey but reinforces the importance of persistence and the cumulative effect of these steps. Each small victory builds upon the last, gradually leading you to reclaim your health and well-being.

PETER McDONALD

Food 4 Families Project

Clontarf, Queensland, 4019

Australia

CONTENTS

Introduction

Unmasking the Hidden Pandemic: Hypothyroidism

In a world where medical advancements have brought hope to countless lives, a silent epidemic continues to undermine the health of millions: hypothyroidism. Often undiagnosed or misdiagnosed, this underactive thyroid condition quietly wreaks havoc on the lives of those it affects. The hidden nature of this disorder, coupled with the widespread reliance on blood tests that fail to capture the full spectrum of thyroid dysfunction, has left a significant gap in our healthcare system—one that has profound implications for global health.

Hypothyroidism is more than just a thyroid problem; it is a systemic issue that affects every cell, tissue, and organ in the body. When the thyroid gland does not produce enough hormones, the body's metabolism slows down, leading to a range of symptoms that are often dismissed as part of aging or stress. Fatigue, weight gain, depression, and cognitive impairment are just a few of the symptoms that can drastically reduce the quality of life for those affected.

Despite the prevalence of these symptoms, hypothyroidism remains underdiagnosed. The standard approach to diagnosis, which relies heavily on Thyroid Stimulating Hormone (TSH) levels, often fails to identify those who suffer from this condition.

As a result, millions of people are left untreated, struggling with symptoms that could be alleviated with proper diagnosis and treatment.

This book seeks to shed light on the hidden pandemic of hypothyroidism. Drawing on the work of pioneering doctors from the past and present, it aims to provide a comprehensive understanding of the condition, its symptoms, and the limitations of current diagnostic methods. By exploring natural and holistic approaches to managing hypothyroidism, this book empowers readers to take control of their health and find the treatment that works best for them.

In Unmasking the Hidden Pandemic: Hypothyroidism, we will delve into the history of thyroid treatment, uncover the reasons why this condition is often overlooked, and offer practical solutions for those seeking to restore their health. Whether you are newly diagnosed, suspect you have hypothyroidism, or are simply interested in learning more about this pervasive yet often ignored condition, this book will guide you on your journey to better health.

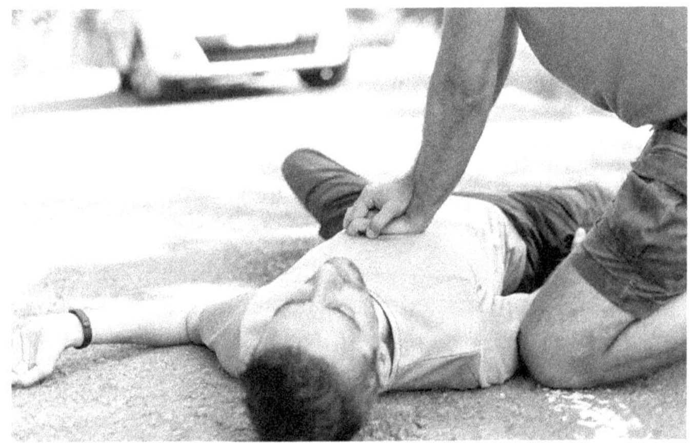

My Easter Sunday Shock: A Sudden Cardiac Arrest

*L*et me briefly share how my near-death experience led to the discovery of my hypothyroidism, underscoring the critical role of preventive medicine. I was fortunate to get a second chance at life, but many may not have that opportunity, which is why understanding the thyroid gland's importance to overall health is so vital.

Easter Sunday 2020 started like any other day at my health and wellness stall at the Mt. Gravatt markets. But that day, my life took an unexpected turn. While chatting with my wife, Alma, and our friend Patsy, I suddenly collapsed and went into cardiac arrest. No warning signs, no symptoms—just a blackout.

Five hours later, I woke up in Princess Alexandra Hospital, confused but feeling surprisingly well.

The story of my collapse is nothing short of miraculous. I was surrounded by quick-thinking heroes: Alma, Patsy, and Claire, an off-duty nurse who appeared out of nowhere to coordinate CPR, and the paramedics. Without their swift and selfless actions, I wouldn't be here today to share my story.

Cayenne Pepper: The Unexpected Lifesaver

Amid the chaos, Alma and Patsy acted swiftly to place cayenne pepper capsules under my tongue. This quick action was crucial in saving my life and preventing brain damage. Dr. Christopher, known as Dr. Cayenne, advocated this practice for heart attack victims. His teachings emphasized the immediate benefits of cayenne on heart health.

Claire, an off-duty nurse, stepped forward to assist Alma and Patsy. She coordinated CPR until the ambulance arrived, about 15 minutes later. I later had the chance to thank her when she revisited the markets.

When the paramedics arrived, I was struggling to breathe. I soon became unconscious, and they used a defibrillator, administering four shocks to revive me. I was in a high-risk condition when I left the markets, but by the time I reached the hospital, ten minutes later, I was back to normal. There was no brain damage — a remarkable outcome.

Cardiac Arrest Despite a Healthy Lifestyle: Uncovering the Hidden Risk

*C*ardiac arrest, unlike a heart attack, is an electrical problem that causes the heart to stop beating. In my case, there was no blockage in my heart—just an electrical malfunction that disrupted my heart rhythm.

So, why did I suffer a cardiac arrest despite being healthy? I've always had normal blood pressure, a balanced diet, and no major health issues. For over 38 years, I've been involved in the health and wellness industry, living a lifestyle that supports good health. Yet, this sudden event caught me completely off guard.

My cardiac arrest was a stark reminder that health can be unpredictable. Despite living a healthy lifestyle, I faced a life-threatening situation without warning. The quick actions of those around me, and the unexpected intervention of cayenne pepper, saved my life. This experience has made me even more grateful for every day and more aware of the delicate balance of health.

My story emphasizes the importance of quick action and awareness. Patsy and Alma's immediate response with cayenne pepper, nurse, Claires, coordination of CPR, and the paramedics' swift intervention were all critical. Knowing such life-saving techniques can make a difference in emergencies.

Dr. Cayenne's Wisdom

Dr. Christopher, affectionately known as Dr. Cayenne, once said, "In 35 years of practice, and working with people and teaching, I have never on house calls lost one heart attack patient and the reason is, whenever I go in— if they are still breathing— I pour down them a cup of cayenne tea (a teaspoon of cayenne in a cup of hot water), and within minutes they are up and around). This is one of the fastest-acting aids we could ever give to the heart because it feeds the heart immediately. Warm tea is faster working than tablets, capsules, and cold tea because the warm tea opens up the cell structure- -makes it expand and accept the cayenne that much faster, and it goes directly to the heart, through the artery system, and feeds it in powerful food. "

Reflecting on that day, I realize how many guardian angels I had. From Alma and Patsy's quick thinking to nurse, Claire's timely intervention, and the paramedics' relentless efforts— I am here today because of their collective actions.

Five hours after the incident, when I awoke from my slumber, my wife mentioned her lips were on fire from the cayenne pepper during mouth-to-mouth resuscitation. Interestingly, I didn't taste the cayenne at all, as my body must have absorbed it to combat the cardiac arrest. This recovery, without any brain damage or physical impairment, is truly remarkable and underscores the body's resilience and the effectiveness of quick medical intervention.

Understanding the Difference Between Cardiac Arrest and a Heart Attack

Cardiac arrest is an electrical issue, while a heart attack is a circulation problem. Despite no blockages, my heart's electrical system short-circuited, causing my collapse. This can happen to anyone, regardless of their health status.

Surviving the Odds: The Miracle of My Recovery

When the cardiac attack story was explained to me, I felt incredibly blessed to be alive. Without any brain damage or physical impairment, I realized I was in the right place at the right time. Had I been anywhere else that day—walking alone or even asleep in bed—I might not be here today to tell my story. It's a sobering thought.

As a healthy person, I was baffled by my cardiac arrest. I needed to understand why it happened. Before this incident, I had no heart symptoms, no blockages, and my blood pressure was always normal. Since leaving the hospital in April 2020, my daily blood pressure readings averaged 114/76, my heartbeat was 72, and my weight remained steady. I led a healthy lifestyle, ate a balanced diet, and took health supplements. So why now?

The Thyroid Gland: The Hidden Pandemic's Master Regulator

During my week-long hospital stay, tests revealed the unexpected culprit: my thyroid. I had an extreme case of hypothyroidism, known as myxedema. To say I was surprised is an understatement. Despite numerous blood tests over the years, my thyroid issue had never been detected. It turns out that because I hadn't specifically requested a thyroid test, it wasn't automatically included.

Considering thyroid issues affect 30-40% of the population and has done so for decades, you would think a thyroid test would be standard with every blood test. This is why hypothyroidism is often called the hidden pandemic—many people are unaware they have it and don't get tested for it.

A paper published in the Journal of the American Medical Association nearly 60 years ago asserted that low thyroid function or hypothyroidism is the most common disease among those visiting a doctor's office. Unfortunately, it is also the most frequently missed diagnosis.

Dr. Robert Thompson, in his book "The Calcium Lie 2," estimates that 80-90 percent of the population has some degree of hypothyroidism. Many patients are mislabeled as hypochondriacs and treated for depression when the underlying issue is low thyroid function.

As far back as 1933, Dr O.P Kimbal, after a 10-year study, five years carried out at the famed, Cleveland clinic, and five years in private practice, was reporting that" In practice of medicine today, no more important condition is encountered, or so often unrecognized as hypothyroidism".

Dr Arnold Jackson, reported in the Journal of the American Medical Association to the fact that " Hypothyroidism is the most frequent chronic affliction and at the same time the most often overlooked condition affecting people. My statement is based upon an experience of thirty-seven years in diagnosing and treating thousands of these cases seen at the Mayo and Jackson clinics".

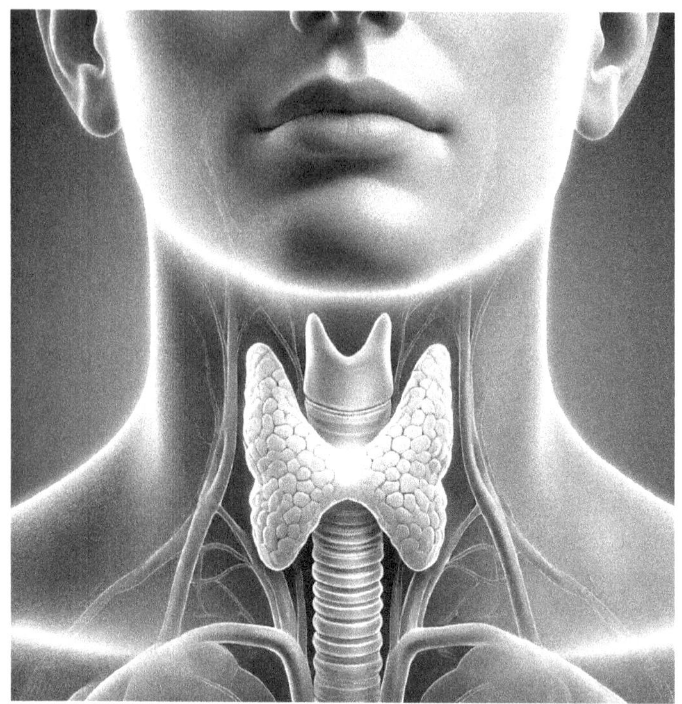

Recognizing the Silent Symptoms of Hypothyroidism

I had never realized the critical role the thyroid gland plays in overall health. My experience underscored the importance of understanding and monitoring thyroid health, which can significantly impact various bodily functions.

The thyroid gland is a small, butterfly-shaped gland located in front of the throat, below the Adam's apple, and above the breastbone. If you wore a tie, it would be where the knot lies. Weighing less than 28 grams, it is considered a master gland. It plays a critical role in your body's overall function. It regulates the body's metabolism by producing and releasing thyroid hormones—primarily thyroxine (T4) and triiodothyronine (T3)—into the bloodstream. These hormones affect nearly every organ in the body and control many vital functions, including:

- **Energy Production:** Determining the rate at which your cells produce energy from nutrients.
- **Heat Generation:** Regulating body temperature.
- **Growth and Development:** Crucial for normal growth and brain development in children.
- **Heart Function:** Influencing heart rate and the strength of heart contractions.
- **Metabolism of Fats and Carbohydrates:** Affecting weight and energy levels.

The Pituitary Gland's Role

The pituitary gland at the base of the brain controls hormone production in your body by making Thyroid Stimulating Hormone (TSH), which tells the thyroid gland how much T4 and T3 to produce. A basal temperature test with a reading below 36.5 degrees Celsius (97.8 F usually indicates an underactive thyroid or hypothyroidism.

If everything is working properly, your body produces the correct amounts of thyroid hormones, which control the metabolism of every cell in your body. However, imbalances can lead to significant health issues. Poor thyroid function has been linked to conditions such as fibromyalgia, irritable bowel disease, vitiligo, gum disease, infertility in women, and other autoimmune diseases.

In his book "Hypothyroidism: The Unsuspected Illness," Dr. Broda Barnes illustrates the critical role of the thyroid. He describes removing the thyroid glands from baby rabbits, which led to their fur becoming dry and falling out, weight lagging, repeated infections, and early death. Administering thyroid hormone to some rabbits resulted in a quick recovery, highlighting the thyroid's vital role.

**Recognizing the Silent Symptoms of Hypothyroidism
*(continued)***

The symptoms of hypothyroidism can vary widely based on the severity of hormone deficiency.

Common symptoms include:

- Fatigue and sluggishness
- Increased sensitivity to cold
- Constipation
- Dry skin
- Weight gain
- Puffy face
- Hoarseness
- Muscle weakness
- Elevated blood cholesterol levels
- Muscle aches, tenderness, and stiffness
- Joint pain, stiffness, or swelling
- Heavier or irregular menstrual periods
- Thinning hair
- Slowed heart rate
- Depression
- Impaired memory

Causes of Hypothyroidism

Hypothyroidism occurs when your thyroid gland, a crucial part of your endocrine system, can't produce enough hormones to keep your body functioning optimally. This hormone deficiency results from a lack of stimulation by the pituitary gland, the master gland, located at the base of the brain that secretes the thyroid-stimulating hormone (TSH).

Several factors can cause hypothyroidism, including Hashimoto's Thyroiditis, an autoimmune disease where the immune system mistakenly attacks the thyroid gland. It is the most common cause of hypothyroidism, leading to the thyroid stopping hormone production. This condition occurs more frequently in women than men.

Myxedema is a severe, life-threatening form of hypothyroidism. Low levels of intracellular T3 can lead to cardiogenic shock, heart attacks, stroke, respiratory depression, hypothermia, and coma. This condition has a high mortality rate and requires immediate medical attention.

Other factors, that can cause hypothyroidism are:

- **Allopathic treatment** (drugs and medication) for hypothyroidism, such as radioactive iodine (levothyroxine) or surgery aimed at reducing thyroid hormone levels, can sometimes lead to hypothyroidism.
- **Thyroid surgery:** Removing part or all of the thyroid gland.
- **Radiation therapy:** Radiation used to treat cancers of the head, neck, or chest can affect the thyroid gland.
- **Medications:** Certain drugs can impact thyroid hormone production.
- **Iodine deficiency:** Iodine is essential for thyroid hormone production. Deficiency is a common cause of hypothyroidism in areas where iodine intake is insufficient.
- **Congenital issues:** Some babies are born with a thyroid gland that is not fully developed or functional.

Effective Diagnosis and Treatment: Managing Hypothyroidism

Modern medicine's treatment for hypothyroidism typically involves the daily use of the synthetic thyroid hormone levothyroxine. While this medication can help restore adequate hormone levels, it comes with certain precautions. It is not advisable for individuals who have had heart disease, cardiac arrest, or a stroke, as it can potentially trigger the very symptoms they are trying to avoid. Most people with hypothyroidism will need to continue this treatment for life, and doctors may increase the dosage over time based on regular TSH monitoring.

So instead of finding the cause of the problem, most doctors perform a blood test and prescribe levothyroxine as the medication and keep increasing the dosage of levothyroxine until the blood test shows an increased TSH level. This is a symptomatic solution to manage the problem.

The Thyroid Pioneer: Dr Broda Barnes: Groundbreaking Insights

*D*r. Broda Barnes spent 50 years treating hypothyroid individuals. He was an assistant professor of medicine at the University of Illinois. He was the author of four books about thyroid, including the book "Hypothyroidism: The Unsuspected Illness" and published over 100 research papers.

He made the comment that continually raising the levothyroxine level is not the way to go to get a positive outcome. That method is symptomatic, not a long-term healing approach to managing hypothyroidism. When thyroid function is deficient, the gland cannot respond adequately to the stimulus from the pituitary. Then it is necessary to supply a small amount of thyroid hormone from the outside, just as insulin is supplied for the diabetic.

But remember the feedback mechanism. If an excess of thyroid is supplied from the outside, the pituitary gland will get the signal that there is such an excess and will stop its stimulus to the thyroid gland, and thyroid function may be depressed still further. With sufficient excess supplied from the outside, the thyroid may stop putting out any hormone.

In that case, all thyroid is coming from the outside, the body's precise control of thyroid level in the bloodstream is thwarted, and it is possible that the patient may even have too much hormone in the blood and may develop some of the symptoms of hyperthyroidism, such as nervousness, sleeping difficulty, excessive sweating, elevated temperature, and loss of weight.

None of this is necessary. If a small dose is used to begin with and the dose is raised only if necessary, and then gradually, the thyroid gland will continue to function as it has before, its deficiency will be overcome, the feedback mechanism will be maintained intact, and the amount of thyroid in the bloodstream will be kept in the effective narrow range found in people with normal thyroid function. One mistake that has been made in the past has been to start thyroid therapy with excessive amounts.

Holistic Approaches: Non-Drug Treatment for Hypothyroidism

Orthomolecular treatment uses natural substances like vitamins, minerals, and nutrients to help the body heal and function properly, without relying on synthetic drugs. It involves assessing nutritional status through tests to identify deficiencies or imbalances. A personalized plan is created, often including supplements and dietary adjustments to correct these deficiencies. This approach aims to support the body's natural processes, improve overall health, and reduce the need for medications, focusing on long-term nutritional status and toxic element exposure.

Orthomolecular, natural, non-drug treatment for hypothyroidism typically involves daily supplementation of specific nutrients. These include:

- **Lugol's iodine solution or kelp (iodine):** Essential for thyroid function.
- **L-tyrosine:** The body uses this amino acid to produce thyroxine, a crucial thyroid hormone.

- **Selenium:** Important for thyroid gland function and reproduction.

- **Vitamin C complex** (not ascorbic acid): Necessary for the production of thyroid hormones.
- **Chromium:** Supports healthy lipid metabolism.
- **Zinc:** Plays a role in the formation and metabolism of thyroid hormones.
- **Niacin (Vitamin B3)** helps clear plaque and cholesterol from veins and arteries, which can prevent arteriosclerosis (blocked arteries). This is particularly important for people with hypothyroidism, as it is more effective than other medications or drugs for this purpose.

This approach emphasizes the use of natural supplements to support and improve thyroid function.

My Enlightening Journey: Understanding Hypothyroidism

I had taken thyroid issues and hypothyroidism lightly in the past. However, my experience with myxedema—a severe, life-threatening form of hypothyroidism—has shown me the importance of taking thyroid health seriously. Low intracellular T3 can lead to severe depression, stroke, heart failure, cardiac arrest, or coma. My cardiac arrest stemmed from this condition, prompting me to unmask this hidden disease, understand its causes, and find the best solutions to manage my thyroid problem.

My journey has taught me the critical importance of thyroid health. Regular testing and awareness are key to preventing and managing hypothyroidism, ensuring that this hidden pandemic does not go unnoticed and untreated.

Determined to manage my condition effectively, I listened to my doctor's advice on allopathic medications and then conducted my own research. I wanted to make an informed decision on whether to choose medication, drugs (allopathic) or natural supplements (orthomolecular, non-drugs) to address my health condition. My goal was not to treat symptoms temporarily but to find a lasting cure.

In my research, I delved into the past and found many books written by pioneering doctors who successfully managed heart disease and thyroid issues. These doctors dedicated their lives to helping people and documented their findings meticulously. Their research, clinical trials, and case histories on both animals and humans were invaluable.

Lessons from the Past:
The Golden Era of Medical Learning

The 1950s was a period of great learning for doctors. Free from the grip of pharmaceutical companies, they explored both orthomolecular (natural) and allopathic (drugs) medicine to find the best treatments for their patients. They documented their findings, conducted clinical trials, and determined safe dosage limits for managing and healing diseases and infections.

These historical medical books are priceless. They provide a comprehensive view of treatment options, combining modern and past remedies to help make informed decisions about health. Remember, your health is your wealth, and good health cannot be bought. Choose wisely, as many medical procedures cannot be reversed.

Over time, pharmaceutical companies gained the upper hand, and many doctors stopped experimenting with natural medicine. This shift led to fewer books being written about natural alternatives, and allopathic remedies became the norm for almost all health issues, even if they were not the best option for healing. We only need to look at the state of the health of our country to see that the solution hasn't worked. We have a health crisis on our hands which continues to worsen.

Empowering Health Through Knowledge: A Holistic Approach

The books and writings of past and present eminent doctors provided me with sufficient information to manage my condition naturally. They offered insights into how to avoid medications and drugs that could be detrimental to my quality of life and overall health. Reading these books felt like having a consultation with the best doctors, guiding me through my journey with hypothyroidism.

Health remedies change over time, and not always for the better. In today's world of quick fixes, it's crucial to look at the root causes of health issues rather than just treating symptoms. My journey with hypothyroidism and heart disease has taught me the importance of holistic health and the value of natural remedies.

Reflecting on old writings, I discovered that many doctors concluded that low thyroid function was a common factor in the illnesses of many patients. Today, thyroid issues like hypothyroidism remain hidden enemies, often undetected by doctors.

Unseen Threat: The Overlooked Impact of Hypothyroidism

*D*espite the medical industry's aim to improve the diagnosis and treatment of hypothyroidism, heart, and other diseases, it sometimes neglects effective treatments discovered by renowned doctors in the past. This oversight can result in negative outcomes and misdiagnoses, hindering the healing of many current health issues.

Our eminent doctors of the past understood the connection between hypothyroidism, heart disease, and other conditions. They discovered these facts decades ago. They discovered that hypothyroidism, diabetes, tuberculosis, and heart disease all have one thing in common, Atherosclerosis, blocked arteries. Heart disease is the major cause of death amongst people throughout the world today, and Atherosclerosis, blocked arteries, and Atherosclerosis, according to Dr. William Parsons Jr., is responsible for nearly all cardiovascular disease, death, and disability.

Atherosclerosis (blocked arteries) is another hidden enemy; it leads to reduced or blocked blood flow. It is one of the major causes of heart disease, strokes, and cardiac arrest. Effective management of atherosclerosis is crucial for preventing health issues like hypothyroidism, diabetes, tuberculosis, and heart disease.

According to Dr. Robert Thompson, hypothyroidism is simple to diagnose. However, patients often spend years seeking a doctor who will confirm the obvious diagnosis. Modern medicine's fixation on blood tests with falsely expanded normal values, rather than good patient care, reliable histories, laboratory tests, hair tissue mineral analysis (HTMA), and basal body temperatures, has led to the underdiagnosis of this debilitating condition. This is why hypothyroidism is called the hidden pandemic—it goes unrecognized and untreated.

In his book, "The Calcium Lie 2," Dr. Robert Thompson gives a more understanding account of other underlying problems that affect the thyroid and are associated with hypothyroidism. He explains the 5 types of hypothyroidism that exist, something that no other doctor has mentioned to me.

 He found thyroid hormone resistance is beyond epidemic level; it is at a pandemic level and is directly related to excess dietary calcium. The problem is much worse today because most doctors will simply take a TSH (thyroid-stimulating test) blood test and pronounce that your thyroid is fine based on outdated testing procedures and reference levels that are often normal, even when you show all the classic signs of a low thyroid function (hypothyroidism).

The Connection Between Hypothyroidism and Cardiovascular Health

*D*r. Broda Barnes emphasized the need for comprehensive patient care, including thorough examinations and consideration of thyroid therapy. His 20-year, patient study trial, demonstrated that thyroid treatment could dramatically reduce heart attack incidences. Unfortunately, modern doctors often rely heavily on blood tests and overlook physical symptoms and patient histories, leading to missed diagnoses and inadequate care.

In my quest to better understand hypothyroidism and its potential causes, I delved deeply into the research surrounding heart disease, particularly the pioneering work of doctors like, Dr Broda Barnes, Dr. William Parsons Jr., Dr. Abram Hoffer, Dr. Dimitri Kats,Dr Guy Abrahams, Dr David Brownstein and the findings of the Coronary Drug Project (CDP). Their groundbreaking studies on the use of niacin (vitamin B3) to control cholesterol and prevent serious cardiovascular events like heart attacks and strokes caught my attention for several reasons.

Firstly, hypothyroidism has a well-established link to heart disease. The thyroid gland plays a critical role in regulating metabolism, and when it's underactive, it can lead to high cholesterol levels, increased blood pressure, and other cardiovascular issues. Understanding how niacin could potentially alleviate these risks through its ability to raise HDL ("good" cholesterol) and reduce inflammation provided me with valuable insights into how hypothyroidism might be better managed or even prevented.

Niacin's Crucial Role in Cardiovascular and Thyroid Health

Dr. William Parsons Jr. pioneered the use of niacin (vitamin B3) for cholesterol control in the 1950s. His findings, documented in his book "Cholesterol Control Without Diet," revealed that niacin could remove plaque and cholesterol from veins better than any other treatment. He states that niacin unblocks arteries, and with more widespread use of it, countless lives would be saved by preventing heart attacks, strokes, and cardiac arrest. These serious cardiovascular events then would not disturb or destroy the quality of life for so many people. The need for expensive and dangerous cardiac surgery and other invasive methods of treatment would be lessened, expensive hospitalization reduced, and tremendous expenditures on other cholesterol-control drugs avoided.

The Coronary Drug Project (CDP, 1966-1974) was the first United States nationwide multicenter study of any kind. The CDP was the first study to demonstrate that a drug to reduce blood lipids (fat-like substances) would lessen heart attacks, strokes, and cardiovascular surgery. Of the several drugs studied, only niacin (vitamin B3) produced these benefits.

A survey fifteen years later on the people involved in the initial CDP study found that niacin proved to be the only substance in the study to reduce total deaths as well. More recently, niacin has been demonstrated to reduce injury to the brain after strokes.

The Inkeles and Eisenberg report stated that If patients were routinely placed on the proper diet and niacin (vitamin B3) long before they developed any coronary problems, most if not all coronary bypass operations could be avoided.

In 1981 Dr. Inkeles and Dr. Eisenberg reviewed the evidence relating to coronary artery bypass surgery and lipid levels. Their conclusion was "there is still no consensus that this surgery increases survival. The major problem not resolved by cardiovascular surgery is how to halt the arteriosclerotic process.

If every patient requiring this operation were placed on the proper diet and niacin, following the surgery, the progress of arteriosclerosis would be markedly decreased. The surgeons would be able to show a marked increase in useful longevity. Niacin should be used before and after every coronary bypass surgery. Niacin increases longevity and decreases mortality in patients who have suffered one myocardial infarction.

Surely present-day doctors are aware of this information. That should be a given. Why don't more doctors use niacin (vitamin B3) if they look at health objectively. They do so, because they are not good at niacin. They believe the pharmaceutical remedies instead of the tried and true, and no side effect remedies of the past

Dr. Dimitri Kats on Niacin: A Multifaceted Remedy

*D*r. Dimitri Kats has a PhD in Epidemiology from the University of North Carolina at Chapel Hill, and he also has degrees in Biostatistics and Mathematics. His background includes epidemiology, aging research, biostatistics, longitudinal analysis, and psychometrics. He has written a hypothesis paper "A Potentially Critical Role for Niacin in Immunology?" that has far-reaching implications for not only SARS-CoV2 but also for most modern diseases.

Dr. Dimitri Kats found that flush niacin (vitamin B3) is unsurpassed in preventive and therapeutic medicine, with multifaceted benefits not just for viral infectious disease but all diseases.

Inflammation is the root cause of most modern illnesses. More than 50% of all deaths worldwide are attributed to chronic inflammatory diseases, which include cancer, cardiovascular disease, thyroid, hypothyroidism, dementia, stroke, and diabetes. Alzheimer's, Parkinson's disease, prostate, joint pain, arthritis, Meniere's disease, and many more. Hypothyroidism itself is not an inflammatory disease, but it can result from an inflammatory condition like Hashimoto's thyroiditis.

He found that low HDL was the driving force behind all diseases. HDL (high-density lipoprotein) cholesterol, sometimes called "good" cholesterol, absorbs cholesterol in the blood and carries it back to the liver. The liver then flushes it from the body. When HDL is low, you have inflammation. Flush niacin basically burns out fats, sucks out inflammation, and limits lipolysis. Getting more flush niacin into your body increases HDL and your immune system.

The Coronary Drug Project (CDP) demonstrated that niacin could reduce heart attacks, strokes, and cardiovascular surgeries. Despite this, niacin (vitamin B3) remains underutilized in modern medicine. Increasing awareness and use of niacin could revolutionize the treatment and prevention of many diseases.

Taking Charge: The Power of Knowledge in Managing Hypothyroidism

*M*anaging my condition with natural supplements has been crucial in preventing a recurrence of cardiac arrest. I didn't want a band-aid solution, which would always have me thinking will it happen again. I wanted a lasting change. That's why I chose natural remedies to manage my health issues.

I thoroughly researched my health problem, ensuring that the herbs and supplements I take are based on science, clinical trials, and medical reports, not just ancient practices. This approach respects both modern medicine and the effective natural remedies used by past doctors.

When I read books on the subject of hypothyroidism, written by the likes of Dr. Broda Barnes, Robert Thompson, Dr. Guy Abrahams, Dr. David Brownstein, Dr. Abram Hoffer, Dr. William Parsons, what comes across the pages of those books, very strongly, is the emphasis on patient care, ongoing clinical trials and meticulous records of each patient and case histories, and over long periods of time.

Modern Diagnostic Hurdles in Hypothyroidism

Dr. Robert Thompson, author of the book "The Calcium Lie 2", is highly critical of the modern approach to diagnosing and treating hypothyroidism. According to him, the basic problem that traditional medicine has with diagnosing hypothyroidism is the so-called "normal range" confirming the obvious diagnosis. That's because modern medicine has become so fixated on blood tests with falsely expanded normal values instead of good patient care and reliable patient histories. Lab tests, hair analysis tests and basal body temperature data. They are essential, but the physician who conducts them is extremely rare. TSH (thyroid stimulating hormone) is far too high.

Many patients with TSH's of greater than 2.0 (not 4.5) have classic symptoms and signs of hypothyroidism. So, if your TSH is above 2.0 there is a strong chance your thyroid gland is not working properly.

There are a significant number of individuals who have a TSH even below the new 1.5 reference range mentioned above, but their Free T3 (and possibly the Free T4 as well) will be below normal. These are cases of secondary or tertiary hypothyroidism, so, TSH alone is not an accurate test of all forms of hypothyroidism, only primary hypothyroidism.

In his book "The calcium lie 2" Dr Robert Thompsons, comments on managing hypothyroidism, are as follows" thyroid disease should be considered a disorder of production, or a disorder of function, or a combination of both". The mainstream medicines bulldog- like determination, to diagnose hypothyroidism, based on one criterion, the TSH has led to the Thyroid stimulating hormone Lie, which has left millions to suffer needlessly.

The Limitations of Blood Tests

Blood tests only show recent or current exposure, offering a snapshot of mineral and heavy metal levels at the time of the test, which can fluctuate throughout the day. If a person is anxious, has medication that affects the body, or food sensitivity, it will provide an inaccurate account of what is actually going on inside the body.

Blood mineral levels are tightly regulated by the body and can fluctuate throughout the day, which means blood tests may not accurately reflect total body stores or chronic exposure.

Blood collection is invasive, may be painful, and requires a healthcare professional to draw the sample.

Hair Tissue Mineral Analysis (HTMA) Testing: A Superior Tool for Long-Term Nutritional Insight

Dr. Robert Thompson mentions in his book " The Calcium lie 2", "in my experience with reliable hair testing mineral analysis (HTMA) testing over the past 30 years, it is clear this one single test has had a greater impact on my patient's health, in the short and long term, than any other laboratory test, known to mankind".

Dr. Robert Thompson suggests the hair tissue mineral analysis (HTMA) should be a part of the diagnosis and treatment of everyone with hypothyroidism, since the disease has become so common. The results help you see accurately what is going on. In reviewing my records, I have found more than 95 percent correlation, between a HTMA result, showing an elevated ratio of calcium to potassium and low basal body temperatures. This confirms that the intracellular calcium/potassium imbalance causes type 2 hypothyroidism.

Hair Tissue Mineral Analysis (HTMA) offers several advantages over traditional blood tests, particularly when it comes to assessing long-term nutritional status and exposure to toxic elements. Hair analysis reflects mineral and heavy metal levels over a longer period (months), providing a more comprehensive picture of long-term nutritional status.

Hair is a valuable medium for detecting levels of minerals and heavy metals over time, as it stores these substances and provides a long-term record.

Additionally, collecting a hair sample is non-invasive and painless, making it easy to obtain without the need for a medical professional.

Nutritional Considerations

I have implemented many of Dr. Robert Thompson's protocols for my hypothyroidism management. He is renowned for his comprehensive approach to managing hypothyroidism. He emphasizes good patient care, thorough clinical trials, and meticulous record-keeping. His strategies involve using various diagnostic tools and treatments, including the basal temperature test and Hair Tissue Mineral Analysis (HTMA), alongside ionic mineral supplements.

Addressing hypothyroidism involves correcting various nutritional deficiencies and imbalances. Dr Thompsons regime includes balanced ionic trace minerals, DHEA, taurine, tyrosine, iodine, copper, selenium, chromium, zinc, and whole food vitamin C complex (not ascorbic acid).

I include Niacin, my favorite vitamin as part of my protocol as well. Rather than take ten different supplements to form my ionic mineral protocol, I take one supplement called Thyroid Health, which includes Kelp (iodine) & bladderwrack (iodine), vitamin C complex (not ascorbic acid), L-tyrosine,L-glutamine, selenium,magnesium citrate, chromium, zinc, cayenne, and niacin B3 (Inositol hexaniacinate), Vitamin B6: Pyridoxine, and Vitamin B12: Cobalamin.

Tracking Progress:
The Importance of Daily Monitoring

Since my cardiac arrest in April 2020, I've been diligently tracking, and recording my basal temperature, blood pressure, heart rate, and weight almost every day. This comprehensive monitoring allows me to adjust my supplement regimen based on changes in my basal temperature, which is a key indicator of thyroid function. By keeping an eye on my weight, I can identify which foods may not align with my hypothyroidism management plan. Additionally, regular checks of my blood pressure and heart rate help me stay informed about my heart health.

Basal Temperature Testing: A Key Tool in Thyroid Management

*B*asal temperature testing is a simple, yet highly effective method for assessing thyroid function, particularly when diagnosing and managing hypothyroidism. The test involves measuring your body's lowest resting temperature, typically first thing in the morning before any physical activity, food, or drink, which can influence the reading.

Basal temperature testing is used because it provides an indirect but reliable indication of your thyroid gland's activity. The thyroid gland plays a critical role in regulating metabolism and body temperature. When the thyroid is underactive (a condition known as hypothyroidism), it often results in lower-than-normal body temperature.

By regularly monitoring basal temperature, individuals and healthcare providers can gain insights into the thyroid's performance, helping to determine if the gland is functioning optimally or if there are signs of imbalance.

How the Basal Temperature Test Works

Basal temperature testing is a simple and effective method to detect subtle changes in thyroid function that standard blood tests may overlook. It can be done daily in the comfort of your home, giving you consistent insight into your thyroid health. By regularly monitoring your temperature, you can make timely adjustments to your supplements, supporting your thyroid's natural healing process.

In contrast, traditional tests like TSH (thyroid-stimulating hormone) are typically performed every three to four months. This approach leaves gaps in tracking your thyroid's daily function, making it harder to address issues promptly. It's a reactive, short-term fix that often leads to ongoing reliance on medication, rather than helping the thyroid regain its full function naturally.

Basal temperature testing, on the other hand, can highlight issues by showing consistently low temperatures, a sign of an underactive thyroid. This method is especially useful for those who suspect thyroid problems but have normal lab results.

Additionally, daily basal temperature tracking is a great tool for assessing the effectiveness of thyroid treatments. By monitoring temperature fluctuations, individuals can adjust their supplements or medications to optimize thyroid function, aiming to maintain a healthy body temperature between 36.5°C to 37.0°C (97.8°F to 98.6°F).

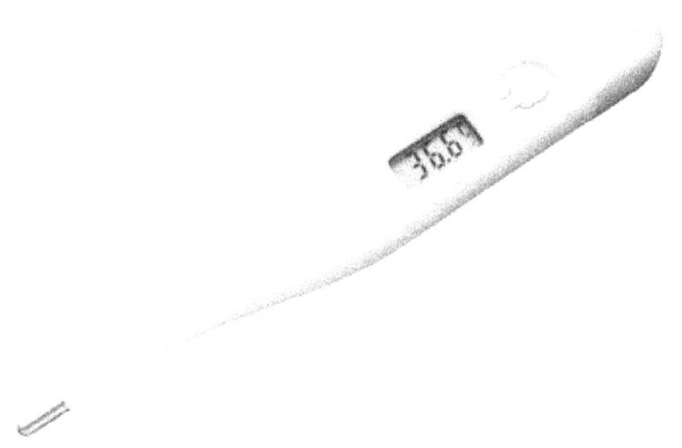

1. **Preparation**

- The test is best performed first thing in the morning, immediately after waking up, and before getting out of bed. Before any physical activity, eating, drinking, or even speaking. This is because the body's temperature is at its lowest after a full night's rest, and any activity can raise the temperature and affect the accuracy of the test.
- It's important to use a reliable digital thermometer or a basal body thermometer, which is more sensitive to small changes in temperature compared to regular thermometers.

2. **Measurement**

- Upon waking, take your temperature by placing the thermometer under your tongue (or using an armpit measurement if directed by your healthcare provider).
- Keep the thermometer in place until it beeps, indicating the reading is complete. For some basal body thermometers, this might take a few minutes.

3. **Recording**

- Record the temperature immediately, ideally in a logbook or a health tracking app. It's crucial to do this consistently at the same time every morning, before getting out of bed, to ensure accuracy.

Interpreting the Results

Monitoring my basal temperature has proven particularly valuable in managing my hypothyroidism. The basal temperature test reveals whether my thyroid is functioning properly.

A normal basal body temperature typically falls between 36.5 to 37.0 degrees Celsius (97.8 to 98.6 degrees Fahrenheit). If my temperature consistently measures below this range, it may indicate an underactive thyroid, or hypothyroidism. It signals the need to adjust supplementation to correct the imbalance.

Conversely, consistently higher temperatures, though less commonly tracked with this method, could point to an overactive thyroid, known as hyperthyroidism.

My Protocol for Managing and Improving My Hypothyroidism

To manage my hypothyroidism, I chose to avoid conventional treatments like levothyroxine and instead sought out natural remedies. I delved into the methods used by pioneering doctors, focusing on holistic health and natural supplements. My regimen includes hair tissue mineral analysis (HTMA), daily basal body temperature testing, and taking a balanced blend of ionic trace minerals such as L-tyrosine,L-glutamine, iodine, copper, selenium, chromium, zinc, Vitamin B6 & B12 and a whole food vitamin C complex (not ascorbic acid). To simplify my protocol, I use a supplement called Thyroid Health, which combines these essential elements in one capsule.

I was initially prescribed levothyroxine for my hypothyroidism, but after researching its potential side effects—which can include heart attack (chest pain, shortness of breath), heart failure (extreme tiredness, shortness of breath), and irregular heart rhythm (very fast heart rate)—I decided against taking it. The very issues I was trying to protect, like my heart health and avoiding irregular heart rhythms, were the same issues that levothyroxine could potentially worsen. So, taking levothyroxine was never an option for me.

Given the seriousness of hypothyroidism, I needed an alternative approach. As I mentioned before, I was not comfortable with the idea of taking levothyroxine for life, especially considering the side effects and the lack of personalized care from the endocrinologists I visited. They relied heavily on blood tests to measure thyroid function and believed increasing the dosage of levothyroxine was the solution.

Dr. Broda Barnes, in his book "Hypothyroidism: The Unsuspected Illness," highlights a striking paradox: "It may seem almost incredible that scientists can sit quietly on earth and follow the activity of the heart of a man walking on the moon and yet have so much difficulty in measuring the amount of thyroid hormone necessary for health and in developing effective and reliable tests to determine when thyroid function is inadequate. That's why hypothyroidism is called the hidden enemy; it's not recognized or detected in the first place. It's like a snake hidden in your body: silent, unseen, but capable of striking at any moment."

My research led me to the methods used by many respected doctors of the past for treating hypothyroidism. Their protocol, which predates the use of levothyroxine and amiodarone, involved Lugol's iodine and tyrosine. When taken together, these two elements perform the same function as levothyroxine but without the side effects. That's the approach I decided to take.

What Does L-Tyrosine Do for the Thyroid?

L- Tyrosine, an amino acid, is vital for proper thyroid function. It plays a crucial role in the production of thyroxine, a key thyroid hormone. Thyroxine, the main hormone released into the bloodstream by the thyroid gland, helps regulate metabolism and control the levels of T3 and T4 thyroid hormones. Without sufficient L-Tyrosine, the thyroid gland cannot produce adequate amounts of T4 and T3, leading to potential thyroid dysfunction.

The Role of L-Tyrosine in Thyroid Hormone Production

L- Tyrosine serves as a building block for thyroid hormones. The thyroid gland first absorbs iodine from food. Then, thyroid peroxidase (TPO) oxidizes this iodine into its active form. These active iodine molecules then bind to the tyrosine in thyroglobulin, a protein produced by the thyroid gland. This combination forms thyroid hormone precursors, monoiodotyrosine (T1) and diiodotyrosine (T2). T1 and T2 subsequently combine to create triiodothyronine (T3) and thyroxine (T4), the primary thyroid hormones essential for regulating metabolic processes throughout the body.

The Importance of Thyroxine

Producing enough thyroxine is crucial for preventing symptoms of an underactive thyroid (hypothyroidism). Hypothyroidism can lead to a sluggish metabolism, tiredness, sensitivity to cold, weight gain, constipation, moodiness, and weakness. Historically, doctors used tyrosine as a remedy for hypothyroidism before the advent of medications like levothyroxine and amiodarone. Tyrosine, especially when combined with iodine, has shown a high success rate in treating hypothyroidism.

The Benefits of Iodine and L-Tyrosine

The combination of Lugol's iodine and L-Tyrosine can have a remarkable effect on energy levels. Personally, since incorporating iodine and L-Tyrosine into my routine, I've experienced a significant boost in energy. Previously, as an early riser between 4 and 5 am, I often felt tired in the afternoons and needed a power nap. However, since taking iodine and L-Tyrosine, I can breeze through the afternoon without needing a nap. This improvement in energy levels is particularly impressive considering fatigue and tiredness are common symptoms of hypothyroidism.

L-Tyrosine and iodine together can significantly enhance thyroid function, improving overall energy and reducing symptoms of hypothyroidism. This natural approach highlights the importance of supporting thyroid health with the right nutrients.

L-Tyrosine Dosage for Thyroid Health

The appropriate dosage of **L-tyrosine** in conjunction with iodine for thyroid support can vary depending on individual needs and health conditions. Both L-tyrosine and iodine are essential for the production of thyroid hormones, particularly T3 (triiodothyronine) and T4 (thyroxine), which help regulate metabolism and energy levels.

Here are some general guidelines:

- **Typical dosage:** The common dosage for L-tyrosine supplements ranges from **500 mg to 2,000 mg per day**. For thyroid support, many recommendations fall in the range of **500 mg to 1,000 mg daily**, often divided into two doses (morning and midday) to support the body's natural hormone production.
- **Starting slow:** It's often suggested to start with a lower dose and monitor how your body responds, particularly if you are combining it with iodine.

Iodine Dosage for Thyroid Health

*I*odine is essential for the synthesis of thyroid hormones, but too much can be harmful, especially for those with thyroid issues. The recommended daily allowance (RDA) for iodine in most adults is 150 mcg (micrograms) per day.

Higher doses (up to 200–300 mcg per day) may be used for people with mild iodine deficiency but should be done under medical supervision.

Combining L-Tyrosine and Iodine

Balancing the two: Since both L-tyrosine and iodine are needed for thyroid hormone production, combining them in moderation can support thyroid function, especially in people with hypothyroidism or mild thyroid hormone deficiencies.

Monitoring thyroid function: If you're taking both supplements to support your thyroid, regular monitoring of your thyroid hormone levels (TSH, T3, T4) is recommended to ensure you're getting the right balance and to avoid over-supplementation, which can lead to hyperthyroidism. That's why daily readings of your temperature, using the basal temperature test, is so important for monitoring your supplement intake.

The number of drops that provide 150 mcg of iodine depends on the concentration of the iodine solution you are using.

Here's how you can calculate it:

Lugol's Iodine Solution

1. Lugol's Iodine Solution (2% or 5% Solution)

In a **2%** Lugol's iodine solution, 1 drop contains approximately **2.5 mg of iodine**. To get **150 mcg (0.15 mg)**, you would take a fraction of a drop (about 1/**16 th of a drop**).

In a Lugol's **5%** iodine solution, 1 drop contains approximately **6.25 mg of iodine**. Similarly, **150 mcg** is a small fraction of a drop, around **1/40 th of a drop**.

Since these amounts are hard to measure practically, it's best to use an iodine supplement specifically designed to provide smaller, more accurate doses of iodine, such as iodine capsules or tablets.

Kelp and Bladderwrack Supplements for Iodine

2. Kelp Supplements for Iodine

Kelp is a natural source of iodine, and the iodine content in kelp supplements can vary widely depending on the brand and concentration.

- A typical **kelp supplement** might provide **150 mcg to 225 mcg of iodine per capsule**. If you're aiming for 150 mcg of iodine, you can take one standard capsule, depending on the label's listed iodine content.

Bladderwrack also contains iodine but in lower concentrations compared to kelp. This may make it a gentler option for those looking to avoid excessive iodine intake.

- Bladderwrack has a broader spectrum of nutrients. In addition to iodine, it is rich in **fucoidan**, a compound with anti-inflammatory and antioxidant properties. Fucoidan is not as prevalent in kelp, so bladderwrack might offer more benefits for immune health and inflammation.

Both bladderwrack and kelp contain essential minerals like calcium, magnesium, and potassium, which are beneficial for overall health.

Potential Health Benefits of Kelp and Bladderwrack

3. Potential Health Benefits

- **Kelp** is commonly used as a natural iodine supplement for thyroid support.

- **Bladderwrack** has traditionally been used not only for thyroid health but also for its potential benefits in reducing inflammation, promoting skin health, and improving digestion. Some research suggests that bladderwrack may be beneficial in managing arthritis symptoms due to its anti-inflammatory properties.

Unlocking the Thyroid: How Vitamin C Supports Hormone Production

Another important vitamin for thyroid stimulating hormone production, is vitamin C, particularly in combination with Liposomal Vitamin C, which excels in absorption, In his book "the calcium lie 2" Dr. Robert Thompson mentions, that, thyroid hormones cannot be produced by the thyroid gland without the vitamin C molecule.

Most type 1 hypothyroidism is probably related to chronic C deficiency. Vitamin C regenerates selenoproteins essential for thyroid health, as well as facilitating copper utilization, both necessary for the formation of thyroid hormone. Therefore, the combination of C deficiency and selenium deficiency should be an exact recipe for developing type 1 hypothyroidism (failure of hormone production).

My Daily Supplementation for Optimal Thyroid Health

I've had to navigate my journey to manage hypothyroidism and strengthen my heart largely on my own. Along the way, I've been guided by the work of renowned doctors, both from the past and present, who specialize in thyroid health. Through trial and error, I've experimented with different supplements and dosages to find what works best for my body.

Our body is its own greatest healer—it knows what it needs better than anyone. When given the right nutrition and tools, it can heal itself in its own time and order of priority. After much experimentation with varying dosages, I've come to follow the wisdom of some of the most respected doctors from the past, focusing on providing my body with only the minimal external supplements needed to support its natural healing of my hypothyroidism.

Supporting My Hypothyroidism Naturally

I'm currently following a protocol designed to support my thyroid gland, which in turn should help improve the production of the thyroid hormones T4 (inactive) and T3 (active). These are the two main hormones produced by the thyroid. I'm hoping that my next thyroid blood test and hair analysis will show if this approach is working, and my basal temperature is operating at around 36.5 and up to 37.0 degrees Celsius (97.8 to 98.6 degrees Fahrenheit).

My Protocol to Support the Thyroid Gland

I'm maintaining my iodine intake with 4 drops of Lugol's solution in the morning and 2 drops in the evening. Additionally, I'm incorporating more iodine-rich foods. I've increased my L-tyrosine intake to 2 capsules twice a day and am eating more foods rich in tyrosine, such as chicken, turkey, and almonds, to support thyroid hormone production.

These are some of the other natural supplements I use to help manage hypothyroidism naturally by supporting thyroid hormone production, reducing inflammation, and addressing the root causes of thyroid dysfunction.

Selenium is essential for converting T4 into the active T3 hormone. My selenium dosage is one capsule per day, and I have added more selenium-rich foods like Brazil nuts, fish, and eggs to my diet.

L-Glutamine supports hypothyroidism by improving gut health, boosting immune function, reducing inflammation, and enhancing energy and muscle strength. I'm taking 2 capsules.

Niacin (Vitamin B3) supports energy production and improves circulation, which positively impacts thyroid function and overall metabolic health. It's my favorite vitamin because of its versatility—it's a true multitasker.

Niacin enhances overall health and wellness throughout the body in numerous beneficial ways. I'm taking 1 capsule of non-flushing niacin, 4 times per day and include more niacin rich foods like fish, poultry and fortified grains, in my meals.

Zinc is crucial for thyroid hormone synthesis. I'm taking 1 capsule of Zinc per day and including more zinc rich foods like oysters, pumpkin seeds, and nuts in my meals.

Magnesium Citrate is important for regulating the thyroid-pituitary axis and is involved in numerous enzymatic reactions that support thyroid health.

I'm taking 1 capsule of Magnesium Citrate, twice per day and including more magnesium rich foods, like, leafy green vegetables, nuts, seeds, and whole grains in my meals.

Chromium plays a supportive role in thyroid health by helping regulate blood sugar levels, which can become imbalanced in people with thyroid issues.

Vitamin B12 is crucial for energy production and cellular metabolism, which are processes directly influenced by thyroid hormones. Vitamin B12 deficiency is common in people with autoimmune thyroid conditions like Hashimoto's thyroiditis or Graves' disease.

Vitamin B6 is involved in the production of neurotransmitters and hormones, including those that regulate the thyroid.It supports the conversion of thyroid hormone T4 (thyroxine) into the more active form T3 (triiodothyronine), essential for proper metabolism.

Vitamin D supports the immune system and helps regulate thyroid function. Deficiency in vitamin D is often linked to autoimmune thyroid diseases.Sources: Vitamin D supplements, sunlight exposure, fatty fish, and fortified foods.

It may seem like I'm taking a lot of supplements to manage my thyroid issues, but I've had to navigate much of this journey on my own. I've been guided by the work of renowned doctors from the past who specialized in thyroid health. Through trial and error, I've experimented with different supplements and dosages to discover what works best for me.

Although I take various supplements, I've found that the Thyroid Health supplement contains many of the key ingredients I need. It includes kelp and bladderwrack (both natural sources of iodine), vitamin C, Vitamin B6 and B12, L-tyrosine, L-glutamine, selenium, chromium, cayenne, and zinc. For those seeking a simpler approach, taking two capsules twice a day provides similar benefits to taking multiple supplements separately, making it a much more convenient option.

Many respected doctors from the past came to a similar conclusion: "You can't expect good results from a single large dose of supplements. Instead, it's essential to divide the doses and take them consistently throughout the day, so that the blood levels remain steady."

The biggest problem with people taking natural (orthomolecular) remedies for any health issue is, they don't take enough supplements to see if they work. Dr. Richard A Passwater in his classic health book "Supernutrition" suggests a simple and nontechnical method to determine what amounts of vitamins you personally need to take for optimum health. Wisely, no prescriptive list is given, "no one size fits all" approach is offered. Dr Passwater suggests a slow start, then increase your own vitamin dosage in two-week intervals, until peak health has been achieved. Essentially you take the smallest amounts of supplements that give the greatest result. No one has ever died from taking vitamins.

Despite concerns, the 38th annual report (2020) from the American Association of Poison Control Centers (AAPCC) revealed zero deaths from vitamins.

Supporting data System from the most recent information collected by the U.S. National Poison Data system (in table 22B, Page 1476-1478) at the very end of the full report, published in Clinical Toxicology.

The AAPCC reports zero deaths, from any vitamins at all, which reassured me as I experimented with my health management strategy.

Avoid Environmental Toxins:

I try to reduce exposure to toxins like fluoride, chlorine, and bromine, which can interfere with thyroid function.

Stay Hydrated: Celtic Sea Salt Intake

Just before breakfast, I take 1/5 teaspoon of Celtic Sea salt in a cup of water. I need to constantly remind myself to drink at least 5 glasses of water per day, in conjunction with small quantities of Celtic Sea salt with each glass of water. This aids digestion and helps balance my electrolytes.

I also add 5 sprays of 3% hydrogen peroxide in every glass of water or lemon drink (5-6 glasses per day) I drink, to kill off bad bacteria in the gut, which is where all disease starts.

One of the most noticeable and irritating symptoms of my hypothyroidism is a persistent hoarse voice, particularly after speaking a lot, or eating acid-forming foods. This forms a mucus, phlegm build up in the throat area, which is very uncomfortable and irritating. To alleviate this, I take one tablespoon of Swedish Bitters tincture mixed with one tablespoon of water after every meal, which has been effective in clearing my throat and reducing mucus, and phlegm buildup.

Another effective protocol, I have implemented to reduce the mucus and phlegm buildup in my throat, is, focusing on supplements that contain Quercetin as a key ingredient. I'm currently taking two capsules each of licorice root, moringa leaf, stinging nettle, and quercetin root, once daily. Already, I'm noticing a significant reduction in the mucus and phlegm.

Exercise:

I make sure to include regular, moderate exercise in my routine, as it helps balance hormones and supports the HPT axis.

Dr. Broda Barnes' Approach to Managing Hypothyroidism

Dr. Broda Barnes, a pioneer in thyroid health, and author of the book "Hypo-thyroidism: The Unsuspected Illness" spent over 50 years researching and treating hypothyroidism. His approach emphasizes the critical role of the thyroid in overall health and advocates for thorough, patient-centered care.

His personalized approach to hypothyroidism emphasized addressing the underlying causes rather than just managing symptoms. He was critical of relying solely on **levothyroxine**, viewing it as a symptomatic treatment that did not support long-term healing. He believed that giving the thyroid less external help allowed for a better chance of recovery, and healing, over time.

Key components of his approach include:

1. **Basal Body Temperature Test:** Dr. Barnes championed the use of basal body temperature as a diagnostic tool, considering consistently low temperatures a sign of hypothyroidism.
2. **Natural Desiccated Thyroid (NDT):** He favored NDT over synthetic hormones like levothyroxine because NDT provides both T3 and T4, which more closely mimic natural thyroid function.
3. **Symptom-Based Diagnosis:** Dr. Barnes focused on patient symptoms—such as fatigue, weight gain, and cold intolerance—over blood tests like TSH levels, believing they provided a more accurate diagnosis of hypothyroidism.
4. **Preventing Heart Disease:** Dr. Barnes also linked untreated hypothyroidism to an increased risk of **heart disease**, believing that proper thyroid treatment could reduce this risk.

In summary, Dr. Barnes emphasized **natural thyroid support**, symptom-based diagnosis, and minimizing external hormone interventions to promote long-term healing and overall health.

Dr. Robert Thompson's Strategies for Managing Hypothyroidism

Basal Temperature Test

- **Monitor Your Metabolism:** Dr. Thompson, voted one of the best doctors in the USA, in the 1990s, and author of the book "The Calcium Lie 2", recommends using the basal temperature test as a simple, yet effective way to gauge your thyroid function. By tracking your body temperature first thing in the morning, you can gain insights into your metabolic rate.

Hair Tissue Mineral Analysis (HTMA)

- **Unlocking Mineral Imbalances:** Hair Tissue mineral analysis (HTMA) testing is a cornerstone of Dr. Thompson's approach. It reveals vital information about mineral deficiencies and imbalances, which are crucial for understanding thyroid health.

Adrenal Health and Hypothyroidism: The Hidden Connection

Adrenal Fatigue and Thyroid Issues

- **Overlapping Symptoms:** Many symptoms of adrenal fatigue, such as fatigue, weight gain, and depression, are identical to those of hypothyroidism. This overlap can complicate diagnosis and treatment.

Addressing Adrenal Insufficiency

- The Sodium Solution: Dr. Thompson treats adrenal insufficiency with increased sodium intake, specifically grey sea salt. This helps restore the sodium/potassium membrane electrical potential (MEP), crucial for adrenal and overall metabolic health.

Essential Supplements for Adrenal and Thyroid Health

- **Balanced Minerals:** Dr. Thompson emphasizes the importance of balanced ionic trace minerals.
- **Key Supplements:** His regimen includes DHEA, taurine, tyrosine, iodine, copper, and whole food vitamin C complex (not ascorbic acid). These supplements help support adrenal and thyroid function.
- **Methyl Donors and Cortisol:** He also recommends MSM and, in some cases, low-dose bioidentical cortisol to support hormone balance and overall health.

Dr. David Brownstein's Personalized Approach to Hypothyroidism

Individualized Treatment Plans

No "One-Size-Fits-All": Dr. Brownstein, in his book "Overcoming Thyroid Disorders," stresses the importance of treating each patient as a unique individual.

His personalized approach to hypothyroidism emphasizes treating the root causes of thyroid dysfunction through a holistic, integrative method.

His approach focuses on individualized care, patient education, and empowering patients to take charge of their health.

Key components include:

- **Iodine Supplementation:** He stresses iodine as crucial for thyroid function, often recommending supplements to correct deficiencies.
- **Natural Desiccated Thyroid (NDT):** Dr. Brownstein prefers NDT over synthetic hormones, as it more closely mimics natural thyroid hormone balance.

- **Nutritional Support:** Addressing deficiencies in iodine, selenium, chromium, zinc, magnesium, and vitamin D, which are vital for thyroid health.
- **Avoiding Goitrogens:** He advises limiting foods like raw cruciferous vegetables that may interfere with thyroid function.
- **Detoxification:** Reducing exposure to toxins like bromine and fluoride that compete with iodine, often using detox protocols.
- **Adrenal Support:** Recognizing the thyroid-adrenal connection, he supports adrenal health with lifestyle changes and supplements.
- **Comprehensive Testing:** He uses a range of tests, including Free T3, Free T4, and thyroid antibodies, beyond just TSH.
- **Diet and Lifestyle:** Dr. Brownstein advocates for a nutrient-dense diet, stress management, regular exercise, and sleep to improve thyroid health.

The Role of Hair Tissue Mineral Analysis (HTMA) in Diagnosis and Treatment

I'm pleased with the progress I've made in managing my

hypothyroidism and heart issues. I generally feel strong both mentally and physically. However, my basal temperature still fluctuates, some mornings. In short, my basal temperature, which I take each morning, before getting out of bed, is not registering at 36.5 and up to 37.0 degrees Celsius (97.8 to 98.6 degrees Fahrenheit), it is slightly below that reading. This has led me to look deeper into what might be affecting my thyroid, including how my adrenal glands might be involved.

I wanted to find the underlying problem causing the inconsistent basal temperature readings to support my natural supplement protocol, and when I continued my research on the subject, particularly the work of Dr. Robert Thompson, I believe I uncovered a hidden enemy, that needs to be dealt with and balanced, before any real healing takes place. The potassium to sodium, and the magnesium to sodium imbalance ratio, in the body, are those hidden enemies.

Understanding Sodium and Potassium Balance: in Adrenal Fatigue and Hypothyroidism

The balance between sodium and potassium in the body is incredibly important, especially for managing conditions like adrenal fatigue and hypothyroidism. Potassium is mostly inside the cells, helping with fluid balance, nerve, and muscle function, and eliminating waste from the cells. Sodium, on the other hand, is found outside the cells and plays a key role in maintaining your blood pressure and regulating salt and water balance.

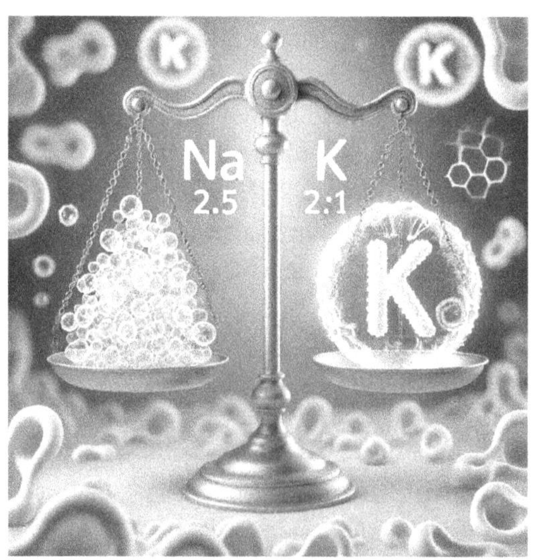

The ideal sodium to potassium ratio for everyone should be 2.5 to 1. This balance is crucial because it is a measurement of your life energy and vitality. This balance supports essential bodily functions, from nerve transmission to muscle contraction, and is fundamental to feeling energetic and healthy. When this ratio is optimized, it's often reflected in better physical and mental well-being, which is why it's sometimes referred to as a measure of "life energy and vitality".

This ratio is significant because it reflects the balance between adrenal and thyroid activity. A ratio higher or lower than this optimal range may indicate imbalances. If it is less the pituitary gland needs some additional outside help to fix the problem. If one or the other electrolytes, sodium, or potassium, becomes too high or low, it could result in severe illness, or even death (scientific nutrition 2020). This is why it needs to be monitored and adjusted, regularly, to understand and address this imbalance.

My hair analysis (HTMA) results showed that my sodium to potassium ratio is exactly 2.5 to 1, which is ideal. However, both sodium and potassium levels are three times higher than average. This might suggest that my adrenal glands are under stress, causing my body to release more sodium and potassium into my hair.

The sodium to potassium ratio does differ with a blood test.The sodium is supposed to be much higher than potassium. If your sodium level is 139 mmol/L and potassium level 4.6 mmol/L, the ratio is Approximately 30.2:1. This ratio is within the normal range for blood serum.

Based on his 25 years of hair tissue mineral analysis (HTMA) and basal temperature testing, Dr Thompson concluded that many of the symptoms of adrenal fatigue, adrenal insufficiency, and suppression are identical to the symptoms of hypothyroidism.

Adrenal insufficiency, or suppression, is much more common than conventional medicine acknowledges, and it often goes hand in hand with other metabolic malfunctions like insulin resistance and thyroid hormone resistance, autoimmune disease, allergies, and chronic illness.

The correct balance of potassium to sodium helps reawaken and correct the sodium/potassium membrane electrical potential (MEP) and helps restore the digestion of proteins carrying the essential amino acids needed to restore the adrenal hormone levels' function and the mineral balance.

Dr. Thompson treats adrenal insufficiency with increased sodium intake (grey sea salt) and recommends HTMA testing to identify and address the root cause of thyroid and adrenal issues.

Understanding the Hypothalamus-Pituitary-Thyroid (HPT) Axis and Thyroid Support

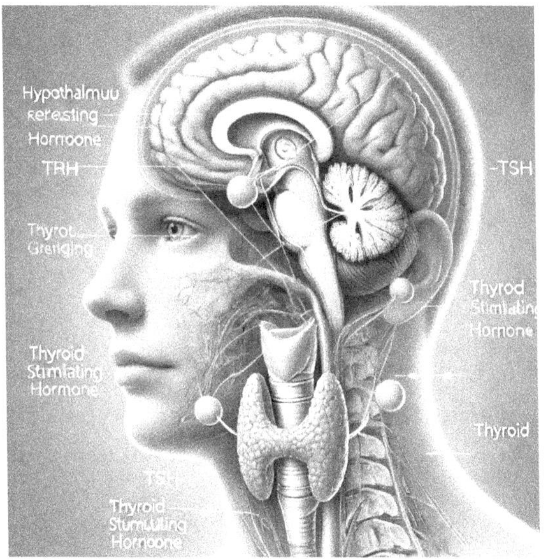

*R*ealizing that my thyroid alone isn't the only factor, in balancing my thyroid, I began looking at the glands that support it, particularly focusing on the hypothalamus-pituitary- thyroid (HPT) axis. This is a crucial system in the body that controls the production and release of thyroid hormones.

The hypothalamus-pituitary-thyroid (HPT) axis is a pathway involving the hypothalamus, pituitary gland, and thyroid gland. Here's a simplified breakdown:

1. **Hypothalamus:** This part of the brain acts as the control center. It releases thyrotropin-releasing hormone (TRH) when the body needs more thyroid hormones.
2. **Pituitary Gland:** In response to TRH, the pituitary gland releases thyroid-stimulating hormone (TSH) into the bloodstream. TSH tells the thyroid to produce thyroid hormones.
3. **Thyroid Gland:** The thyroid produces two main hormones, T4 (inactive) and T3 (active), in response to TSH. T4 is converted into T3 in various tissues throughout the body.
4. **Feedback Loop:** When there are enough thyroid hormones in the blood, they signal the hypothalamus and pituitary to reduce the production of TRH and TSH, maintaining balance.

The hypothalamus-pituitary-thyroid (HPT) axis is essential for regulating metabolism, responding to stress, controlling body temperature, and supporting growth and development.

Supporting the Pituitary Gland Naturally

My current protocol for managing my Hypothyroidism is working well, however, if my adrenal glands are under stress, causing my body to release more sodium and potassium into my hair. I needed to look at reducing this imbalance, and these are the areas I targeted to help support my pituitary gland better.

Manage Stress Levels

Although I don't consider myself an anxious person, I've noticed that as I age, I'm not managing stress as well as I used to. To better handle stress and support my thyroid, pituitary, and adrenal glands, I've found ashwagandha and star anise supplements to be particularly beneficial, because of their calming effect on the whole body.

To enhance their effects, I intake two capsules of each, of these adaptogenic herbs,per day. In addition, I practice yoga regularly, which helps lower cortisol levels and further manage stress.

Balanced Diet

I have placed a lot more emphasis on my diet, and what I eat. I follow a nutrient-rich diet, full of antioxidants, healthy fats, and essential vitamins. My diet is a blend of Mediterranean-MIND (Intervention for Neurodegenerative Delay, and Macrobiotic styles, which I believe supports my overall endocrine health.

I weigh and record my weight daily. This allows me to keep an eye on my weight, so I can identify which foods may not align with my hypothyroidism management plan. Additionally, daily checks of my blood pressure and heart rate help me stay informed about my heart health.

Sleep and Circadian Rhythm

I prioritize getting 7-9 hours of quality sleep each night and sometimes take a power nap during the day. The "Sleep the Night Away" supplement, which includes the ingredients, Ashwagandha root, Valerian root,Star anise, Magnesium Citrate, helps me maintain a consistent sleep pattern without disrupting my nighttime rest. Good sleep is the key to maintaining hormone balance and supporting the pituitary gland.

Summary

*I*n the four years since my cardiac arrest, I have been under the hospital's care to manage my health. During this time, I've had five echocardiograms, seven blood tests (including tests to monitor my thyroid), and six hospital visits for routine check-ups. The echocardiogram, which uses ultrasound to create images of my heart's muscle and valves, has shown that my heart is functioning well with a normal rhythm.

I am grateful for the excellent follow-up care provided by the hospital, which allows me to monitor my progress while using natural remedies to manage my condition. My doctor's overall assessment is positive, stating that everything is functioning as expected. While my thyroid is improving, there's still room for progress, which I continue to work on daily.

Embarking on my journey to find alternative remedies for my hypothyroidism and heart health was both challenging and enlightening, especially in the face of opposition from conventional medical advice.

When I first set out to explore alternative treatments for my hypothyroidism and heart health, I faced significant skepticism and resistance from many healthcare professionals. The conventional approach centered around allopathic medications like levothyroxine, it seemed to be the only accepted solution. However, the potential side effects and lifelong dependency on these drugs prompted me to seek other options.

Determined to find a more holistic and sustainable approach, I delved into extensive research. I started by reading books and studies by pioneering doctors from the past who had successfully managed thyroid and heart conditions with natural remedies. This exploration led me to discover the powerful benefits of Lugol's Iodine, L-Tyrosine, and niacin.

The journey was not easy. The medical community's heavy reliance on pharmaceutical solutions often overshadowed the valuable insights and effective treatments documented in historical medical practices. Despite this, I persisted, driven by the belief that true healing could be found in understanding and addressing the root causes of my conditions.

The opposition I faced only fueled my determination to find answers. I spent countless hours studying clinical trials, patient case histories, and the meticulous research conducted by doctors during the Golden Era of Medical Learning in the 1950s. These doctors had explored both orthomolecular (natural) and allopathic medicine (drugs) to find the best treatments for their patients, free from the overwhelming influence of pharmaceutical companies.

Through this research, I uncovered a wealth of knowledge that modern medicine often overlooks. I learned that many effective treatments for hypothyroidism and heart health had been forgotten in favor of pharmaceutical solutions.

Reading the works of Dr. Broda Barnes, Dr. Robert Thompson, Dr Abram Hoffer, Dr William Parsons,Dr. Guy Abraham, and Dr. David Brownstein, I realized the critical importance of patient care, ongoing clinical trials, and thorough documentation.

Incorporating these natural remedies into my routine, supported by daily basal temperature monitoring and Hair Tissue Mineral Analysis (HTMA), led to significant improvements in my health. My energy levels increased, and the symptoms of hypothyroidism and heart issues began to diminish.

This journey taught me the value of perseverance and open-mindedness. It showed me that true healing often requires looking beyond conventional wisdom and being willing to explore alternative paths. By combining the timeless insights of past medical pioneers with modern knowledge, I found a holistic approach that addressed the root causes of my conditions and improved my overall well-being.

About the Author

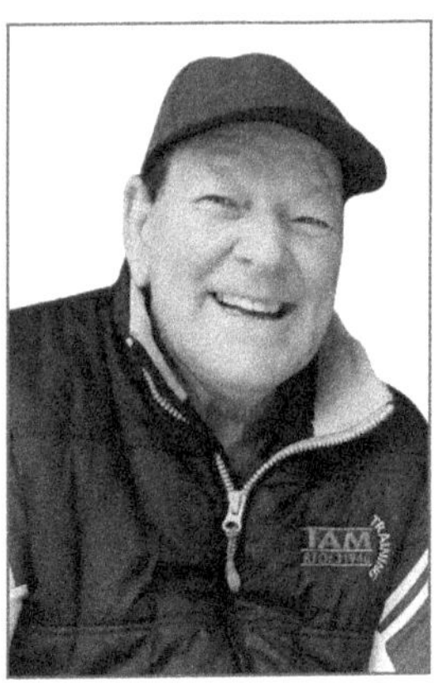

*T*he author of this book, Peter McDonald, is a 3rd generation baker, both his father and grandfather were bakers.

His grandfather Joseph Patrick McDonald opened his first bakery in Mt Kokeby via Beverley, Western Australia in 1903. A further bakery was opened in Beverley in 1907 and during the depression he and Joseph Peter McDonald (Peter's dad) opened a bakery in the mining town of Mt Palmer, Western Australia in 1936, right up until the closure of the town in 1942.

Peter has been involved in the health food industry in Australia for over 38 years, as a distributor, teacher, manufacturer, and retailer. He started teaching sourdough, allergy free, bread baking in 1989 using the unique macrobiotic technique perfected by Jacques deLangre of Celtic Sea salt fame. Jacques deLangre (Phd in biochemistry) from Magalia, California, USA, who researched and taught the lost art of sourdough bread baking for over 35 years.

In 1994, he opened the Celtic Organic Bakery and the Celtic Organic Health Food Store which specialized in whole food, in Alicia St, Southport, Queensland, Australia. The Celtic Bakery specialized in providing allergy-free bread and ran for 10 years. A further whole food store was opened at the Pines shopping center, Elanora, Queensland in 2000.

Celtic Organic Bakery was one of a small number of bakeries in Australia, that milled the organic grain on the premises, providing rancid-free sourdough bread to their customers. The organic grain was freshly milled on the premises and used immediately to make rancid-free sourdough bread. The bread was made with 3 ingredients only, Organic flour, filtered water, and Celtic Sea salt, and without the use of processing aids or any other artificial additives. People with wheat and gluten allergies (not celiacs) were amazed at being able to eat real bread without reacting to any existing allergies or intolerance.

Peter, still bakes organic, whole wheat sourdough bread for his family and friends and continues to provide advice to people on how to make real bread.

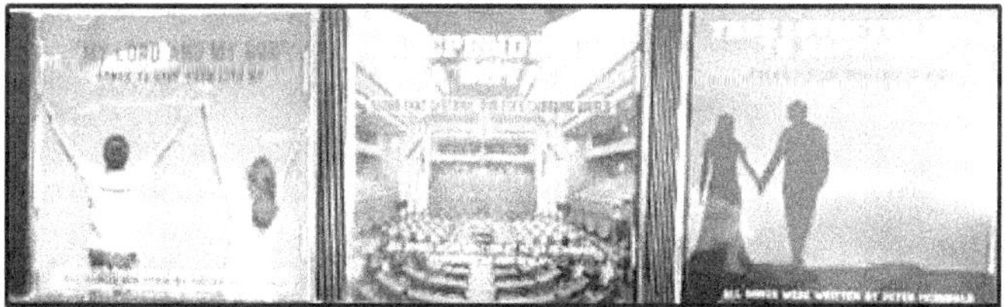

He is a songwriter, his genre is country, folk, pop, protest, and spiritual music, and he has just completed and recorded his tenth album of songs, sung by various artists around the world. He is a scriptwriter and wrote the script and music to the musical "We're Dancing".

His *first book* "**How Cayenne Pepper Saved My Life**" is an account of his own amazing recovery from a cardiac arrest using natural remedies.

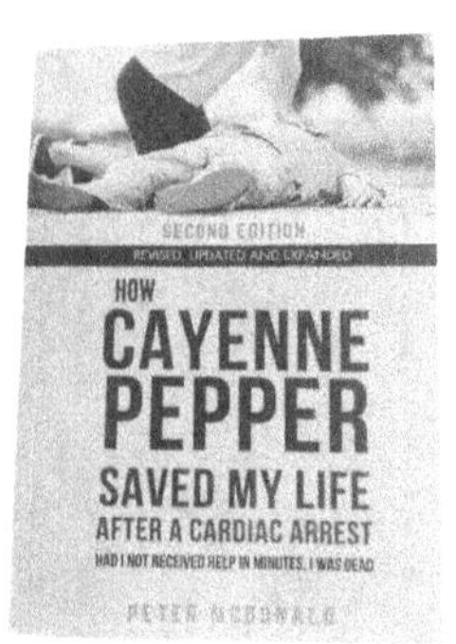

His *second book*, "**Real Bread, Evil Bread**", was 8 years in the making, and it explains the lost

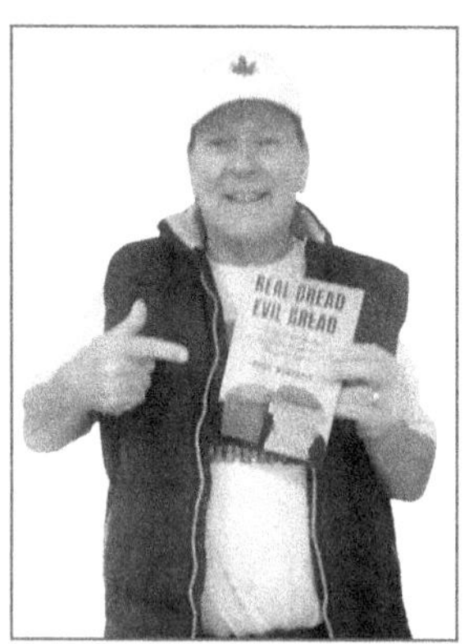

secrets of ancient sourdough and allergy free bread baking. It is a collation of the notes and information passed on from Jacques deLangre PHD (author of the book "Sea Salts Hidden Powers") and Professor Louis Kervran, (author of the book, "Breads Biological Transmutations), as well as his own information and that of many others.

His latest book "**Unmasking the Hidden Pandemic: Hypothyroidism**" is a reflection of his own personal journey with a condition that is often misunderstood and underdiagnosed. The book shares his experiences of navigating traditional medical approaches that didn't fully address his symptoms, leading him to explore alternative, holistic methods that have made a real difference. Through this book, his hope is to shed light on the broader impact of hypothyroidism and offer guidance to others seeking effective ways to manage their health, naturally.

For details on ordering books or song albums
Contact *ganopeter@yahoo.com.au*
www.food4familiesproject.com